THE DIVERTICULITIS GUIDE TO LIVE PAIN FREE

Diverticulitis Diet Plan, Foods to Eat & Avoid, Diagnosis and Tips for Causes, Recovery and Prevention

Nancy Peterson

TABLE OF CONTENT

Introduction

Before the 20th century, it was rare to see anybody with this disease. However, this has become one of the most known health conditions in the West today. Simply put, diverticulitis is a combination of conditions that can affect one's digestive tract.

Diverticulitis is the most serious of the diverticular disease. Diverticulitis is capable of causing very uncomfortable symptoms, which can lead to severe complications for some people.

If this health condition is not treated on time, these serious complications can lead to long-term health challenges.

In this book, I will teach you all you need to know about diverticulitis, causes, tell-tale symptoms, available treatment options and the role that your diet plays in developing or preventing this sickness.

Chapter 1

What is diverticulitis?

Diverticulitis is a type of disease that affects your digestive tract. It is seen as a serious medical challenge that can cause inflammation of the pouches in the linings of your intestine. These inflamed pouches are called the diverticula. They occur when the weak parts of your intestinal wall give way as a result of pressure; this then causes that part of your body to swell out.

Most of the time, the pouches happen in the large intestine, also known as the colon.

Diverticulitis vs. diverticulosis

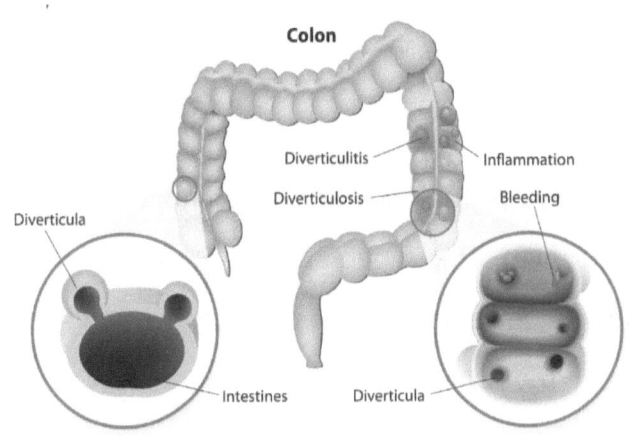

Diverticulosis is a type of diverticula disease that is neither inflamed nor infected. An individual can have diverticula without any inflammation or infection. Diverticulosis is not as serious as the diverticulitis. Most people that have diverticulosis do not experience any symptoms, and researchers confirmed that about 80% of people with diverticulosis do not experience any symptoms. Diverticulosis without any symptom is known as asymptomatic diverticulosis. If you have diverticulosis without experiencing any symptom, you most likely will not need to undergo treatment.

However, there is the remaining 20% who may feel symptoms like bloating and pain in the abdomen. These persons may feel pain in the lower abdomen, particularly in the lower left side of your abdomen. This pain usually occurs when the individual passes stools or eats. You may feel some kind of relief after breaking wind. This condition is known as symptomatic Uncomplicated Diverticular Disease (SUDD).

Other symptoms associated with diverticulosis include:

- Constipation
- Changing bowel habits
- Small amounts of blood in stools
- Diarrhea (very rare)

Research has also shown that about 4% of people with SUDD end up having diverticulitis.

Diverticulitis, on the other hand, can be chronic or acute. In chronic diverticulitis, infection and inflammation may go down, but it never actually clears up. The acute form of diverticulitis may cause one or more severe attacks of inflammation and infection. With time, if left untreated, the swelling may cause pain in the belly, bloating, constipation, diarrhea and thin stool.

Causes of Diverticulitis

The diverticular disease happens when pouches form around your digestive tract, most commonly in your colon (the large intestine). When the diverticular gets infected and inflamed, it becomes diverticulitis. Most times, this happens when feces or food that are not properly digested, blocks the opening of the diverticula.

As at now, scientists have been unable to explain the exact cause of the diverticular disease. However, experts believe that one's environment, as well as multiple genetics, can add to the development of the diverticular disease. Also, as you grow older, your chances of getting diverticulitis increases. The sickness is more common in people who are above the age of 40. Other risk factors are:

- Smoking
- Diet rich in animal fat and low in fiber
- Being overweight
- Not exercising enough
- Taking certain kinds of drugs, including opioids, steroids, and nonsteroidal anti-inflammatories like naproxen or ibuprofen

Symptoms of Diverticulitis

Symptoms of diverticulitis can range from mild to severe. The symptoms may just suddenly appear or may develop slowly over several days.

Possible symptoms of the diverticular disease include:

- Abdominal pain
- Diarrhea
- Bloating
- Constipation

If your condition develops into diverticulitis, you may experience the following symptoms:

- Fever and chills

- Severe or constant pain in the abdomen

- Nausea and vomiting

- Bleeding from the rectum

- Blood in your stool

- Painful urination

- More frequent urination

The most prevalent symptom of diverticulitis is abdominal pain, which will most likely be on the lower-left side of the abdomen. However, this does not mean that you cannot experience the pain on the right side of your stomach.

If you experience any of the symptoms listed above, like seeing blood in your stool or vomiting, it could be a sign of a severe complication caused by diverticulitis. You should contact your doctor immediately.

Chapter 2

Diagnosis of Diverticulitis

Before a doctor can confirm that you have diverticulitis, he or she needs to know if you are experiencing any symptoms, your health history as well as any medications you are currently on.

You doctor will then carry out a physical examination on you to look out for tenderness in your abdomen. If they are not satisfied and need more information, the doctor will then conduct a digital rectal exam to check for masses, rectal bleeding, pain and other problems.

However, note that these symptoms are not unique to diverticulitis alone, as other health conditions can have these same symptoms. To be sure that what you have is diverticulitis, your doctor might request for one or more of the tests listed below:

- Abdominal MRI scan, abdominal ultrasound, abdominal X-ray or abdominal CT scan, to get pictures of your gastrointestinal tract (GI).
- **Stool test,** to look out for infections like Clostridium difficile.
- **Colonoscopy,** to inspect the inside of your GI tract.
- **Blood tests,** for signs of anemia, inflammation, liver or kidney problems.
- **Urine test,** to confirm if there are any infections.
- **Pregnancy test,** to be sure that the patient is not pregnant.
- **Pelvic exam for women,** to check for other gynecological problems.

How to Diagnose Diverticulitis with Colonoscopy

Your doctor might advise you to do a colonoscopy if you have any of the symptoms of diverticulitis. The colonoscopy will be conducted after the severe episode is over.

From this procedure, the medical professional will be able to ascertain if you have diverticulitis or other health conditions that bear a resemblance to diverticulitis, like the Crohn's disease or ulcerative colitis.

To perform the colonoscopy, your doctor will first place you on a sedative to help you stay comfortable. Your doctor will then thread in a flexible scope into the colon and rectum. Through this scope, the doctor will check the inside of your colon, and also collect tissue samples for testing.

In some cases, your doctor may discover that you have diverticula while doing a routine colonoscopy. If the diverticula are not infected, inflamed or causing symptoms, you may not need to undergo treatment.

Complications

For patients that have diverticulitis, results from the tests and examinations conducted will let the doctor know whether your case is complicated or uncomplicated.

Studies show that over 75% of diverticulitis cases are uncomplicated, while the remaining 25% are complicated.

These complications may include:

- **Phlegmon:** this is an infected area that has less confinement than an abscess.
- **Abscess:** a well-enclosed area that is infected and filled with pus. Most times,

antibiotics are administered to dry the pus. But if antibiotics fail, you may need to go through minor surgery to drain the pus.

- **Intestinal perforation:** a hole or tear in the intestinal wall that can let the contents of the colon leak into the abdominal cavity, which can cause infection and inflammation.

- **Fistula:** an abnormal tube or tunnel that connects two parts of your body, like a connection between two different organs or a connection of an organ to the skin. A fistula occurs when infected tissues touch each other, then remain stuck together. In most cases, surgery is needed to remove a fistula.

- **Intestinal obstruction:** a situation where the intestine is blocked, making it impossible for stool to pass through.

Depending on the extent of the blockage, you may need a colon resection or a colostomy. The medical practitioner makes a hole on the side of the abdomen, through which the colon is redirected and connected to an external colostomy bag. The colon is rejoined once it heals completely. There are also rare cases where the doctor may need to create an internal ileoanal pouch.

Risk Factors for Diverticulitis

Age is one of the common risk factors for diverticulitis, as this condition is more common among older adults than youths.

Diverticulitis is more common with men from age 40 and women within the ages 50 to 70. If peradventure, an individual under this age bracket develops the diverticular disease, the chances are that he will have diverticulitis.

Research also shows that young people with diverticulitis have more chances of being admitted at the hospital than the older adults.

Following a review of research published in 2018, other possible risk factors of diverticulitis are:

1. Family history

Two studies carried out showed that genetics play a significant role in diverticular disease. The authors quoted that about 40-50% estimate of the possible risk of the diverticular disease comes from genetics.

2. Low-fiber diet

Some research showed that people who have a low intake of fiber in their diets have a higher chance of having diverticulitis. Other studies also confirmed that there is sufficient connection between fiber diet consumption and Diverticulitis.

3. Low Levels of Vitamin D

A study showed that people that have high levels of vitamin D have a lower chance of having diverticulitis. However, we need more research to explain the connection between vitamin D and diverticulitis.

4. Obesity

Multiple studies have shown that people who have a high body mass and a large waist have increased risk of developing diverticulitis.

There are possibilities that obesity can increase the risk of diverticulitis by changing the balance of bacteria in the gut. Again, we need more research to confirm this.

5. Physical inactivity

Studies have proven that physically active people have a lesser chance of having diverticulitis than people who are not physically active.

6. Use of nonsteroidal anti-inflammatory drugs (NSAIDs)

Constant use of ibuprofen, aspirin or other NSAIDs can increase your risk of getting diverticulitis.

7. Smoking

In the same vein, people who smoke have more chances of getting this disease than people who don't smoke.

Diverticulitis and Alcohol

While we have some studies that show that your alcohol intake may increase the risk of having diverticulitis, other studies have claimed that there is no possible connection between the two.

Your doctor may advise that you reduce your intake of alcohol to avoid any complications. Although consuming alcohol may have no impact on the disease, too much of it can increase your chances of having other serious health issues.

Chapter 3

Treatment for diverticulitis

Your doctor will only recommend treatment after diagnosing the severity of your condition. If the diverticulitis is not complicated, you can treat it at home. Your doctor may either ask that you change your diet or prescribe some medicines that include antibiotics.

However, if you have some complications from diverticulitis, you will need to undergo treatment at the hospital. You may be administered antibiotics and fluids through an intravenous line (IV). You may also need to go through other procedures or even surgery, depending on how complicated your case is.

Changing Diet

To give rest to your digestive system as well as help you to recover speedily, your doctor might ask that you avoid solid food, and follow the liquid diet for some days.

Once the symptoms begin to disappear or get mild, you can then start to eat low fiber foods until there is a total improvement in your condition. Once there is an improvement with your symptoms, your doctor will most likely ask that you add more high fiber foods to your meals and your snacks.

Medication

To reduce the level of discomfort or pain caused by diverticulitis, your doctor may ask that you take over the counter drugs like acetaminophen (Tylenol).

If there is any hint that you may have an infection, your doctor will place you on antibiotics to tackle the infection.

Some of these antibiotics are:

- Amoxicillin
- Metronidazole (Flagyl ER, Flagyl)
- Moxifloxacin

You must finish your prescribed medicines even if you start to feel better after taking the first few doses.

Other procedures

If you have a very complicated case of diverticulitis that cannot be treated via medication and diet change alone, your doctor might probably book you for any of the procedures below:

- **Needle drainage**, here a needle is pierced into the abdomen to take out pus from the abscess.

- **Surgery** is done to either correct a fistula, drain pus from an abscess or remove the parts of the colon that are infected.

Surgery for diverticulitis

If you go through severe cases of diverticulitis that can't be well managed by medication and change of diet, your doctor will have no choice than to recommend you for surgery. Surgery is also used to treat any complication that comes from diverticulitis.

When it comes to treating diverticulitis, we have possible surgeries that can be done. They are:

Bowel Resection With Anastomosis

During this process, the surgeon will remove the parts of your colon that have become infected, then reattach the healthy parts together.

Bowel Resection With Colostomy

For this process, the surgeon will remove all the infected parts of your colon and then attach the end of the healthy part to an opening in the abdomen, referred to as stoma.

Both of these procedures can be done as laparoscopic surgery or open surgery.

How to Prevent Diverticulitis

The world needs more research to know what causes diverticulitis. At the moment, experts believe that several factors may increase one's risk of developing diverticulitis. However, some of these potential risk factors can be reduced when you change your lifestyle.

For example, you may need to do the following:

- Keep a healthy body weight
- Eat meals rich in fiber
- Reduce your intake of saturated fat.
- Take sufficient vitamin D
- Avoid smoking or inhaling smoke from a cigarette

These strategies will not only help to prevent this disease, but will also help with your overall health status.

Chapter 4

Diverticulitis and Your Diet

There isn't an exact certainty on the role of diets in treating diverticulitis. In the same vein, we cannot say that everyone with diverticulitis should avoid these particular foods. However, it is known that there are foods that can either make you feel better or make you feel worse. This confirms that your diet plays a vital role in managing diverticulitis. Your diet is also crucial in ensuring the overall health of the digestive system.

Foods to Eat to Prevent Diverticulitis

Fiber helps promote good digestive health. It keeps the digestive tract clean, promotes good bacteria as well as soften your stool, making it easier to pass. Foods rich in fiber are best eaten by people who do not have diverticulitis but will like to take positive steps to prevent themselves from developing this condition. The recommended daily fiber intake for women is 25 grams, while men should consume 35 grams daily. According to recommendations by the American Academy of Family Physicians, on their website FamilyDoctor.org, men below 50 years should consume 38 grams of fiber daily, while men above fifty years should consume a minimum of 30 grams daily. Women who are below 50 years should consume a minimum of 25 grams of fiber every day, while women above 50 years should consume a minimum of 21 grams of fiber.

It is advisable to increase your fiber intake gradually as a sharp increase in your fiber intake may cause harmful side effects. You also need to drink lots of water to prevent diarrhea, abdominal pain, constipation, gas, and bloating.

Below are some of the fiber-rich foods and their fiber quanity per serving:

- Kidney beans (1/3 cup): 7.9g
- Bran cereal (1/3 cup): 8.6g
- Lentils (½ cup): 7.8g
- Chickpeas (½ cup): 5.3g
- Green peas (½ cup): 4.4g
- Black beans (½ cup): 7.6g
- Pear (1 medium): 5.1g
- Baked beans (½ cup): 5.2g
- Sweet potato, with skin (1 medium): 4.4g
- Soybeans (½ cup): 5.1g
- Bulgur (½ cup): 4.1g
- Mixed vegetables (½ cup): 4g
- Blackberries (½ cup): 3.8g
- Raspberries (½ cup): 4g
- Spinach, cooked (½ cup): 3.5g
- Dates, dried (5 pieces): 3.3g
- Almonds (1 ounce): 3.5g

- Apple (1 medium): 3.3g
- Vegetable or soy patty: 3.4g

Foods that have high fiber count are also rich in vitamins and other nutrients, which is why it is best to get your fiber needs from the foods you consume. However, if you are unable to get all your fiber needs from the food you eat, your doctor may suggest that you add some fiber supplements. Here are some good fiber supplements you may want to get

- **Psyllium.** This fiber option is available in supplements like Konsyl and Metamucil. It is available as a wafer, in granules, as a liquid or as powder

- Chicory root fiber, fructooligosaccharides (FOS), oligofructose, and inulin may help to improve immune function and increase good bacteria (5,6)

- You may also go for **Methylcellulose**-based supplements, like Citrucel, which are available in granular or powder form

Foods to Avoid if You have a Severe Case of Diverticulitis

If you have a serious case of diverticulitis, it is advisable to reduce your consumption of foods rich in fiber for the duration of the sickness. You may also need to avoid solid foods and stick to clear liquid foods, like fruit juices without the pulps, carbonated drinks, water, and gelatin, for a defined time, as advised by your doctor.

Once there is an improvement with your symptoms, your doctor will encourage you to increase your intake of fiber-rich foods. Several studies have proven that high fiber diets can lead to reduced risks of diverticulitis. Other studies have looked at the likely benefits of dietary or fiber supplements for treating diverticular disease. However, there is no certainty of the role of fiber in treating diverticulitis.

Your doctor may also ask you to lower your consumption of red meat, refined grain products, and dairy foods that are rich in fat.

From a large cohort study conducted, it was discovered that people with diets rich in these foods have a high tendency of having diverticulitis than others who eat meals rich in vegetables, fruits, and whole grains.

1. **High-FODMAP foods**

Research has shown that people with irritable bowel syndrome will benefit from diets that have a reduced amount of foods rich in FODMAPs (Fermentable Oligosaccharides, Disaccharides, Monosaccharides, and Polyols). The same applies to people living with diverticulitis.

Examples of food that fall under this category include:

- Certain fruits, such as pears, apples, and plums
- Dairy foods, such as yogurt, milk and ice cream
- Fermented foods like kimchi.
- Cabbage
- Beans
- Garlic and onions
- Brussels sprouts

2. Foods Rich in High Fiber

Foods rich in fiber may benefit diverticulosis patients who do not have serious complications. Eating fiber-rich food as a diverticulosis patient may also stop you from having diverticulitis.

A review of studies done in 2017, on 'diverticulosis and the occurrence of acute diverticulitis,' proved that consuming fiber helps to reduce abdominal symptoms, as well as prevent acute diverticulitis.

But we need to bear in mind that everyone is different, and the fiber needs for each person will differ depending on one's condition and symptoms. If you are experiencing pain or any other symptom, your doctor may advise that you limit the way you consume these fiber-rich foods for some time.

Fiber adds to the stool and may increase colon contractions or peristalsis. This can get quite uncomfortable and painful, especially when having a flare-up.

Avoiding these fiber-rich foods, particularly during a flare-up, can cause your system to rest.

Here are some of the foods rich in fiber that you should avoid during acute diverticulitis:

- Whole grains such as quinoa, brown rice, oats, spelt, amaranth, and bulgur
- Beans and legumes such as chickpeas, navy beans, kidney beans and lentils
- Fruits
- Vegetables

3. Foods High in Sugar and Fat

Studies show that there may be a relationship between foods rich in fat and sugar, and the increase in one's chances of getting diverticulitis. Avoiding foods in this class may help reduce the symptoms of diverticulitis, or even help with total prevention. These foods include:

- Fried foods
- Refined grains
- Red meat
- Full-fat dairy

Other foods to avoid

Previously, doctors advised that people with diverticulitis should avoid eating popcorn, nuts and most seeds. This was with the belief that tiny particles from these foods might stick to the pouches and cause infection. However, most doctors have now moved from this advice as there was no recent study to back up the claim. Some other researches have also advised people with diverticulitis to desist from consuming alcohol.

Foods to Eat with Diverticulitis

There are different treatment and management approaches for individual patients. Your doctor may recommend that you make some specific changes to your diet that will help your condition and reduce your symptoms over time.

If you have a severe case of diverticulitis, your doctor may ask that you follow a clear liquid diet, or a low fiber diet. Let us look at each of these diets.

1. **Low-Fiber Foods**

A low fiber diet, also known as a restricted fiber diet, reduces the amount of high-fiber foods one eats per day. This diet gives rest to the digestive system. A low fiber diet will help with the following:

- Prevent foods that were not well digested from moving through your bowels and intestines.

- Reduce the amount of stool you make.

- Reduce the amount of work done by your digestive system.

- Cause relief with diarrhea, abdominal pain, and other symptoms.

How to Eat (and Recover From) a Low-Fiber Diet

Follow this diet only at your doctor's prescription. The low-fiber diet helps with cramping and diarrhea. Three occurrences may cause a medical practitioner to recommend the low-fiber diet, and these include:

- After some type of surgery

- Before a colonoscopy

- Or in the event of a sudden increase in gut challenges, like diverticulitis.

This diet is restrictive and limits your nutrient consumption, and so, should not be used for weight loss. Following this diet without proper guidance and consultation with your doctor may cause more harm to your body.

Importance of a Low-Fiber Diet

This diet will help with the following conditions:

- Crohn's disease

- Inflammatory bowel disease

- Diverticulitis

- Ulcerative colitis

- Diarrhea

- Constipation

- Abdominal cramps

- Irritation or damage in your digestive tract

- Trouble with digestion

- Narrow bowel caused by tumor

- Recovering from surgeries like ileostomy and colostomy

- After radiation or other treatments that may affect the gastrointestinal tract

What to Eat on A Low-Fiber Diet?

This diet reduces your fiber intake to about 10 to 15 grams daily for both the men and the women. Stick to this diet only for a short time; until your bowel gets better, you recover from surgery, or the diarrhea is gone.

Low-Fiber Foods

- White pasta
- White bread
- White rice
- Low-fiber hot and cold cereal
- Fats like mayonnaise, olive oil, butter and gravy
- Foods made from refined white flour, like pancakes
- Eggs
- Creamy peanut butter

- Well-cooked fresh or canned vegetables in small amounts
- Peeled potatoes
- Dairy products as long as you can tolerate them
- Tender protein sources like tofu, eggs, fish, and chicken

Low-Fiber Fruits

- Bananas
- Watermelon
- Fruit juices that have no pulp
- Honeydew melon
- Peaches
- Canned fruit
- Cantaloupe
- Papayas
- Nectarines
- Plums

Low-Fiber Vegetables

- Canned or well-cooked vegetables without skins or seeds
- Tomato sauces
- Beets
- Carrots
- Asparagus tips
- String beans
- White potatoes without skin
- Lettuce
- Pureed spinach
- Acorn squash without seeds
- Strained vegetable juice
- Zucchini

Before you eat cucumber, ensure to peel off the skin and remove the seed. For the lettuce and zucchini, best to shred the leaves and eat them raw.

Avoid any food that will be hard for your system to handle, like spicy foods, coffee, tea, and alcohol.

Foods to avoid on a Low-Fiber Diet

- Garlic
- Onions
- Bran
- Potatoes that haven't been peeled.
- Cooked or raw cruciferous vegetables
- Dried and raw fruit
- Lentils
- Beans
- Seeds and nuts
- Whole-grain foods
- Brown or wild rice
- Any fried, spicy or tough food
- Tough or processed meat

Some people who followed this diet complained of constipation, so, ensure to take enough fluid to fight against constipation. Always read food labels when shopping, avoid foods that have more than a gram of fiber. If unsure, speak with your dietician or medical practitioner.

Sample Meal Plan for the Low Fiber Diet

Breakfast: Scrambled eggs, white buttered toast with vegetable juice.

Lunch: Tuna salad sandwich on a non-seeded white roll and half of a banana.

Dinner: prepare a piece of broiled salmon that is lightly seasoned, along with mashed potatoes.

2. Clear Liquid Diet

This diet is more restrictive than other diets. Your doctor will only recommend this diet for a specified number of days.

How to Follow a Clear Liquid Diet

A clear liquid diet is a diet made up of transparent liquids like broth, water, juices that have no pulp. The color of the liquid is insignificant, as long as you can see through them, then that is a clear liquid.

All foods seen as liquid or partly liquid at room temperature, are accepted on this diet. Solid foods, on the other hand, are not permitted on this diet.

How does it work?

Most times, your doctor may prescribe this diet before doing some procedures linked to the digestive tract, like the colonoscopies.

You may also be placed on this diet to help relieve you from the stress of several digestive problems like diarrhea, diverticulitis, and Crohn's disease. Your doctor may also recommend this diet after you must have undergone some types of surgery. This is mainly because these liquids are easy to digest, and it helps to clean out your intestinal tract.

The goal of the clear liquid diet is to keep you away from dehydration while giving you enough minerals and vitamins needed for energy. The diet will also help to rest your intestines and stomach.

The foods that you can eat on this diet include:

- Clear broth (fat-free)

- Carbonated sodas like Pepsi, Sprite, and Coca-Cola

- Clear nutritional drinks. E.g. Ensure Clear and Enlive.

- Coffee with no cream or milk

- Clear soups

- Hard candies like peppermint rounds or lemon drops

- Pulp-less juices like White cranberry and apple

- Honey

- Lemonade with no pulp

- Popsicles without fruit pieces or fruit pulp

- Plain gelatin, like Jell-O

- Spot drinks, like vitamin water, Powerade, and Gatorade.

- Tea with no cream or milk

- Strained vegetable or tomato juice

- Water

- Ice chips
- Ice pops with pieces of finely chopped fruit or frozen fruit puree
- Clear electrolyte drinks

If that food is not on this list, please avoid it. For tests like colonoscopies, doctors will advise you do not take clear liquids that have purple or red coloring.

Clear Liquid Diet Meal Plan

This is a sample menu for the clear liquid diet:

Breakfast

- One glass of fruit juice without pulp

- One bowl of gelatin

- One cup of tea or coffee without dairy

- Honey or sugar

Snack

- One glass of fruit juice without pulp

- One bowl of gelatin

Lunch

- A glass of fruit juice without pulp

- A glass of water

- A cup of broth

- One bowl of gelatin

Snack

- One popsicle without pulp

- One cup of tea or coffee without dairy, or one soda

- Honey or sugar

Dinner

- One glass of water or fruit juice without pulp

- A cup of broth

- A bowl of gelatin

- A cup of tea or coffee or tea without milk or cream

- Honey or sugar

Pros and cons of the Clear Liquid Diet

Pros:

- The diet will help you to prepare or recover from surgery, medical test, or other medical procedure.

- It is very easy to follow.

- It is not expensive to follow.

Cons:

- Because it does not have lots of nutrients and calories, you may get hungry or tired.

- It could be boring

Things You Should Know Before You Start a Clear Liquid Diet

If this is prescribed before a colonoscopy, ensure you stay clear of purple or red coloring as this can affect the test imaging.

Inform your doctor if you have diabetes. Diabetic patients are expected to consume a minimum of 200 grams of carb daily, to help them manage their blood sugar level. Always monitor your blood sugar level and switch back to solid food as soon as possible.

Because of the lack of nutrients and calories in the clear liquid diet, do not follow it for more than a few days. You must follow your doctor's advice.

3. High-Fiber Diet

Yes, avoiding foods rich in fiber will provide you relief from some of your symptoms. However, research has shown that constantly consuming high-fiber foods, mixed with plenty of fruits, vegetables, and whole-grain, may cause a reduction in the risk of getting acute diverticulitis.

Fiber helps to soften the body's waste material, which makes it easy for stool to pass through the colon and intestine. This process causes less pressure on the digestive system, and prevent diverticulitis from forming in the body.

The first thing your doctor will recommend if you have diverticulosis, or if you are just recovering from diverticulitis is to switch to the high-fiber diet. For persons who do not normally take foods rich in fiber, it is best to slowly add it to your diet to prevent any harmful side effects.

It is important to your overall health that you eat enough fiber as this will help your body to stay strong and fight off chronic infections.

Fiber-rich foods also help to reduce constipation, help with weight loss and weight maintenance. Eating foods rich in fiber will reduce the level of cholesterol in your body, thereby lowering your risk of heart diseases and diabetes.

These health benefits of fiber may be because of probiotics found in fibers that help with healthy gut bacteria in the human body.

The Institute of Medicine advises that every woman's daily fiber intake should be 25 grams and 38 grams for men.

There are 16 ways to get fiber in your diet.

1. Consume more of whole foods like whole grains, beans, vegetables, and fruits.
2. Add vegetables to your meals, and let it be the first item you eat—especially non-starchy vegetables.
3. Eat Popcorn; this is one of the best snacks you can get.
4. When hungry in between foods, let fruits serve as your snacks.
5. Go for whole grains as against refined Grains. Examples include brown rice, oatmeal, barley, amaranth, bulgur wheat, buckwheat, freekeh, farro, wheat berries, quinoa, and millet.
6. Take Fiber Supplements. These include psyllium, guar fiber, β-glucans, and Glucomannan
7. Eat more Chia Seeds

8. Rather than taking fruit juice, eat the fresh fruits and Vegetables

9. Eat Avocados

10. Snack on seeds and Nuts or Add to Recipes

11. Use high fiber flours to bake

12. Eat Berries

13. Let your diet have plenty legumes

14. Eat your cucumbers, apples, and sweet potatoes with their skin on.

15. Always read labels and go for food rich in high fiber.

16. Let every meal you eat, contain foods high in fiber.

How to Start Eating Fiber Again

Once your digestive system has recovered, you should return to eating foods rich in fiber by slowing introducing small portions of one fiber-rich food per day. If no symptoms occur after 24 hours, then you are free to add the recommended daily intake to your diet.

Your fiber need is based on your sex and age.

	Adults (50 years and below)	Adults over 50 years
Men	38g	30g
Women	25g	21g

Spread your fiber intake, do not eat all in a single meal. The best way to get fiber is by eating your fruits without peeling off the skin, eating whole grains, vegetables, nuts, beans, and seeds

Know Your Fiber

We have two types of fiber:

Soluble fiber: Examples are peas, apples, and beans. They do not irritate the digestive tracks.

Insoluble fiber: they do not completely dissolve in the body. The undigested bits can irritate the intestines. Examples are grains, whole wheat, and raw vegetables.

Other Diets You Should Consider

No matter the diet you are on, you need to drink a minimum of 8 glasses of fluid every day. This will not only help with dehydration, but will also improve the gastrointestinal health.

Consult with your doctor before you make any changes with your diet. Once there is an improvement with your diet, your doctor may ask that you add low fiber foods slowly into your diet. Once all the symptoms of diverticulitis are gone, you can then resume a balanced diet.

Chapter 5: Home Remedies for Diverticulitis

Home remedies for treating diverticulitis mostly has to do with changing your diet. However, we have other options that can help with the symptoms and the health of the digestive systems.

Some studies conducted proved that some strains of probiotics can help to prevent or relieve the symptoms of diverticulitis. However, we need more research to confirm the potential benefits as well as risks in using probiotics to manage diverticulitis.

Some specific supplements or herbs may also be beneficial to digestive health. However, we have very little research supporting the use of herbs to treat diverticulitis.

Home remedies for treating diverticulitis include:

- Liquid diet

- Low-fiber foods

- Over-the-counter medications

- Probiotics

- High fiber foods

- Aloe Vera

- Digestive enzymes

- Herbs like green tea, garlic, ginger and turmeric

- Acupuncture

- Essential oils like lavender oil. These oils should not be taken orally. You can apply on your skin, add to your bathing water or diffuse it.

When to see your doctor if doing Home Treatment

You should contact your doctor if you have the following:

- Excess vomiting

- High fever above 100°F (38°C)

- Rectal bleeding, no matter the amount.

When to go to ER

- If you experience sudden, severe pain in the abdomen.

- If you feel something is blocking the bowel.

- Excess or continuous bleeding from the rectal

Chapter 6: Other Types of Diverticulitis

1. Meckel's Diverticulitis

Although the diverticular disease is mostly common among adults, we have, however, seen rare cases where babies are born with diverticula. Cases like this are known as Meckel's diverticulum. If there is inflammation of the diverticula, this is called Meckel's diverticulitis.

In some cases, you may not notice any effect of the Meckel's diverticulum while the following symptoms may occur in other cases:

- Bleeding from the rectum
- Abdominal pain
- Vomiting
- Nausea
- Bloody stool

If you think your child may have diverticulitis, ensure to see your doctor.

2. Bladder Diverticulitis

Bladder diverticulitis is a condition where pouches form in the lining of the bladder, thereby poking through the weak spots in the wall of the bladder. In some cases, bladder diverticula may occur at birth. In other cases, it may develop much later in life, when your bladder isn't functioning properly, maybe as a result of an injury or illness. Another case that can cause the bladder diverticula is when the bladder outlet is blocked.

A bladder diverticula that becomes inflamed is called bladder diverticulitis. Your doctor may need to prescribe pain medications and antibiotics to treat bladder diverticulitis.

Surgery will come in if the diverticula need to be repaired.

There is also the possibility that having diverticulitis in your colon can affect the bladder. In some severe cases, you may have a fistula between the bladder and the colon, a condition known as a colovesical fistula.

3. Esophageal diverticulitis

You can also have the diverticula in the esophagus. Like the others, this happens when pouches form in the lining of the esophageal.

However, these cases are rare. And if they happen, they take their time to develop slowly over so many years. As they grow, one may begin to notice the following symptoms:

- Pain when swallowing

- Trouble with swallowing
- Bad breath or halitosis
- Regurgitation of saliva and food
- Aspiration pneumonia: this is what happens when you breathe in saliva or food, thereby causing infection of your lungs.
- Pulmonary aspiration: this is when you breathe in regurgitated food or saliva into the lungs.

Your doctor may prescribe pain medications and antibiotics to treat this condition. Surgery may be needed if the diverticula need to be repaired.

Chapter 7: Conclusion

Diverticulitis is popular in the western world. Most of the times, it can be resolved by a temporal change in diet, along with using the right medication.

However, it can be more serious if one encounters some complications. If you have complicated diverticulitis, your doctor will advise you to seek treatment in the hospital. You may have to go through surgery to correct any damage done to the colon.

If you have diverticulitis or have any further questions about this disease, ensure you speak with your doctor as they will know how to treat the disease as well as support your digestive health.

If you were recently diagnosed with diverticulitis, ask your doctor about the food you need and food you should avoid. If you need further guidance, ask your doctor for a dietician you can talk to. You should deal with a professional that has worked with people with diverticulitis.

Also, always be in touch with your doctor regarding your health.

Other Books by Nancy Peterson

- CELIAC/ COELIAC DISEASE AND THE GLUTEN-FREE DIET: The Adult and Children's Guide to Live Pain-Free. https://amzn.to/2O2b8MP

- HERBAL MEDICINE. The Beginner's Guide: Natural Remedies for Healing Common Ailments with Medicinal Herbs https://amzn.to/2toVB8w

- THE GALLBLADDER DIET: Foods to Eat, Causes, Diagnosis, Tips for Recovery & Prevention and Natural Remedies to Cure Gallstones without Surgery https://amzn.to/313cTi6

- CELERY JUICE: The Natural Medicine for Healing Your Body and Weight Loss

(Contains Secret Celery Recipes) https://amzn.to/2tTiISQ

- ALKALINE PLANT-BASED DIET FOR BEGINNERS: Your Complete Guide for Weight Loss, Boost Your Energy, and Cleanse Your Body with the Alkaline Diet. https://amzn.to/3aPZrSX

- LOW CALORIES DIET PLAN: Foods to Eat to Lose Weight and Stay Healthy. Includes 1,200 to 1,700-Calorie Meal Plans https://amzn.to/37vVyk1

www.ingramcontent.com/pod-product-compliance
Lightning Source LLC
Chambersburg PA
CBHW020329290526
45785CB00007B/2970